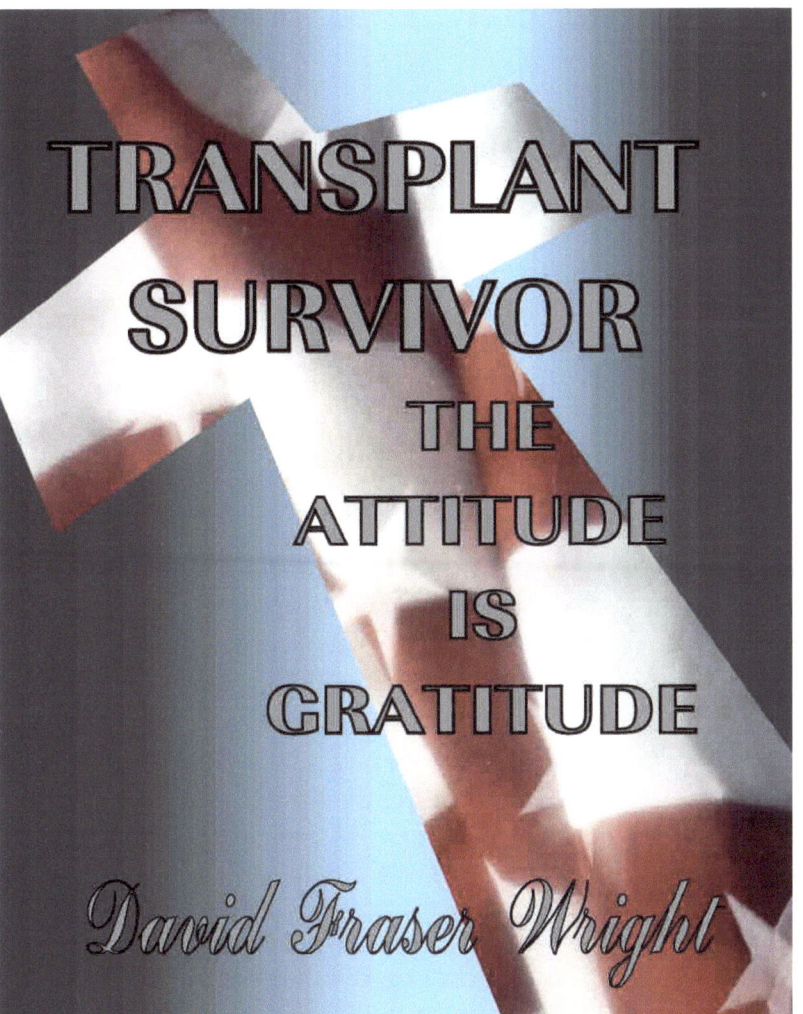

TRANSPLANT SURVIVOR
THE ATTITUDE IS GRATITUDE

by
David Fraser Wright
DavidWrightLIVE.com
All rights reserved.
ISBN-13: 978-1492378778
ISBN-10: 1492378771

No part of this publication may be
reproduced, stored in a retrieval system,
or transmitted by any means -
electronic, mechanical,
photographic (photocopying),
recording, or otherwise -
without prior written permission
from the author.

DEDICATION

Founded in 1984 by Nazih Zuhdi, MD, the
Oklahoma Transplantation Institute was renamed
The INTEGRIS Nazih Zuhdi Transplant Institute in 1999.
It celebrated its 1,000th solid-organ transplant in 1998.
It honors the achievements of many statewide,
as well as national milestones, and medical firsts.
Every day, the INTEGRIS Nazih Zuhdi Transplant Institute
forges new ground in the rapidly developing field of organ
transplantation, finding new ways to offer hope
to those who otherwise may have none –
and who benefit by the INTEGRIS Health Mission:
"to improve the health of the people
and communities we serve."

LEARN MORE ABOUT THEM:
http://www.integristransplant.com

My eternal gratitude is celebrated every day in prayer in
admiration for those who have dedicated their lives to the
service of spirit to their community and humanity.
Those who unselfishly serve have extended the blessing of my
life and those of so many others, and made lives much more
than just tolerable or functional.
I pray for them to enjoy the daily enrichment of their lives
by doing the work of angels.
The gift of one's time, energy, loving care, and
complexity of understanding gives the people they serve
an incalculable gift – *LIFE ITSELF.*
As I read in Corinthians 12, Verses 4 and 5,

"THERE ARE A VARIETY OF GIFTS,
BUT,
THE SAME SPIRIT.
THERE ARE A VARIETY OF SERVICES,
BUT
WE EACH SHARE THE SAME GOD WITHIN."

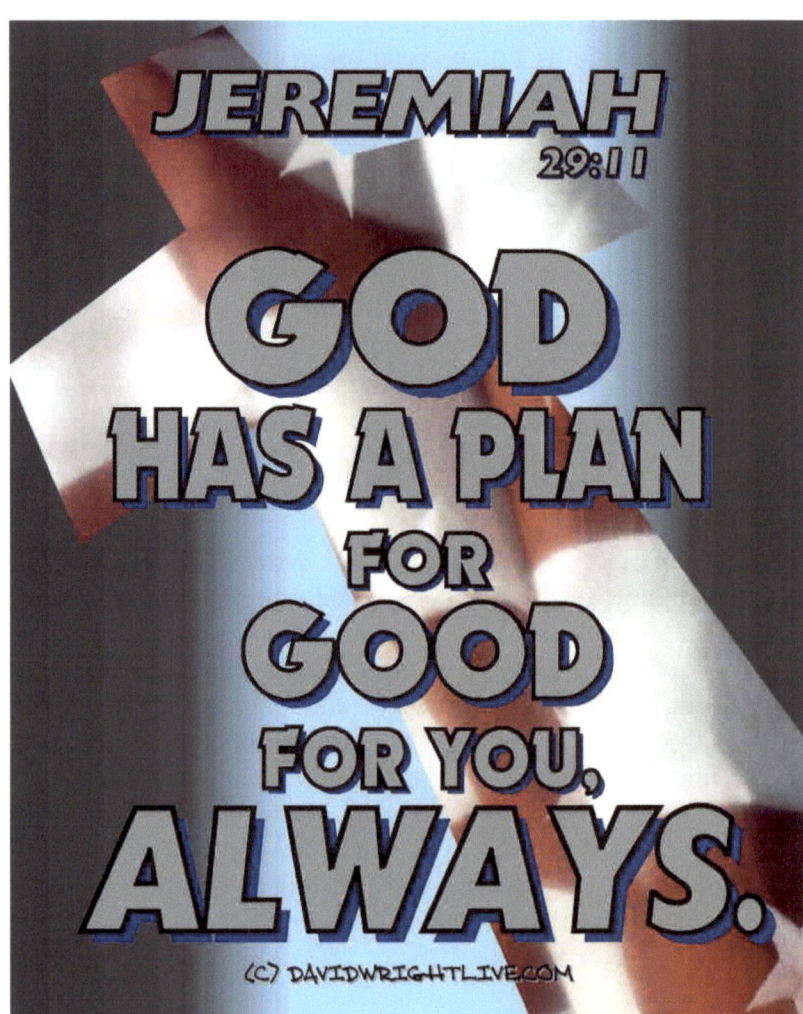

CONTENTS

Having kept a journal of his
thoughts and artwork created over
the 19 year, 7 month, and 7 day journey
from diagnosis of the need for
a life-saving liver transplant,
to being blessed with actually getting it,
David Fraser Wright
has selected ideas, artwork,
and reactions to events,
and presents them to you,
from a year by year compilation -
with the most inspirational
one from each year.

Having survived the transplant,
he celebrates his new life, and
shares how
IT JUST GETS BETTER EVERY DAY.

A GIFT FOR:

_____

FROM:

_____

DIVINE INSPIRATION

This book was inspired by what can only be described as
Divine Intervention over two decades.
Having waited 20 years for a transplant, in a time of terrible
tragedy, a family who I will never know, lost someone near and
dear to them, but had the strength and courage to give me the
opportunity to continue my journey through organ donation.
I pray for them, and for the loved one whose journey ended,
whose nearly perfect match gave me the the chance to
quite literally begin a new life journey of my own.
Over that 20 year period, with a deepening of my faith and
belief system, I enhanced my patience by reading
inspirational works.
One in particular, *"WHAT'S POSSIBLE!," by Author,* and
Creator of the award winning, *DARYNKAGAN.COM,*
DARYN KAGAN gives readers *"TAKEAWAYS,"* such as,
"IS THERE SOMETHING YOU ARE HOLDING ONTO,
WHICH, IF RELEASED, WOULD ACTUALLY
IMPROVE YOUR LIFE?"
Today, I can affirm that by holding onto negatives
from the past, I was removing myself from
the possibilities of a long term positive change.
Understanding this truth, and listening to the Inner Voice
in the sacred silence of meditation and prayer,
I released every concern, and learned everything I
could about what to do to keep myself well enough
to receive the gift of Divine Intervention.
In the book, *"WHAT'S POSSIBLE!,"* I have also learned,
"BY LETTING GO, YOU NOT ONLY IMPROVE YOUR HEALTH
AND LIFESTYLE, BUT YOU PUT YOURSELF IN A POSITION
TO SERVE AND INSPIRE OTHERS WHILE FINDING
NEW JOY AND PURPOSE IN LIFE."
In choosing to take the Leap Of Faith, I let go of all previous
expectations, to let my God Within reveal the possibilities,
and created a vaccuum to bring forth a rush of goodness
and mercy in my life – all in God's Perfect timing.

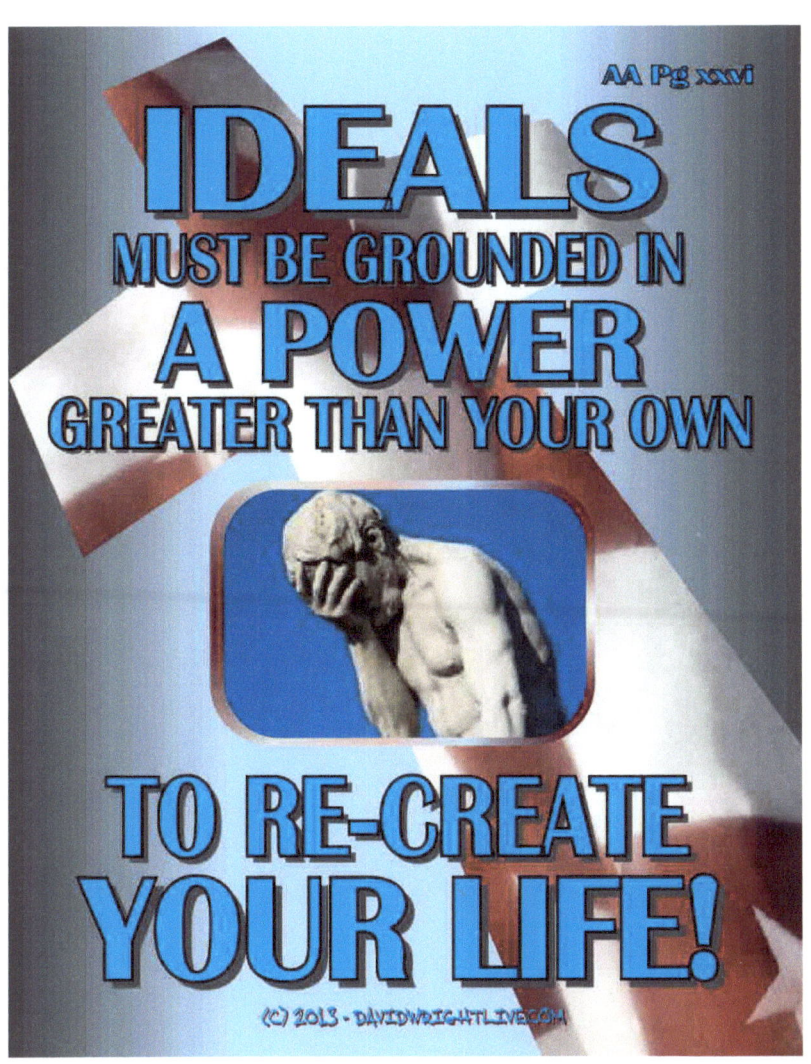

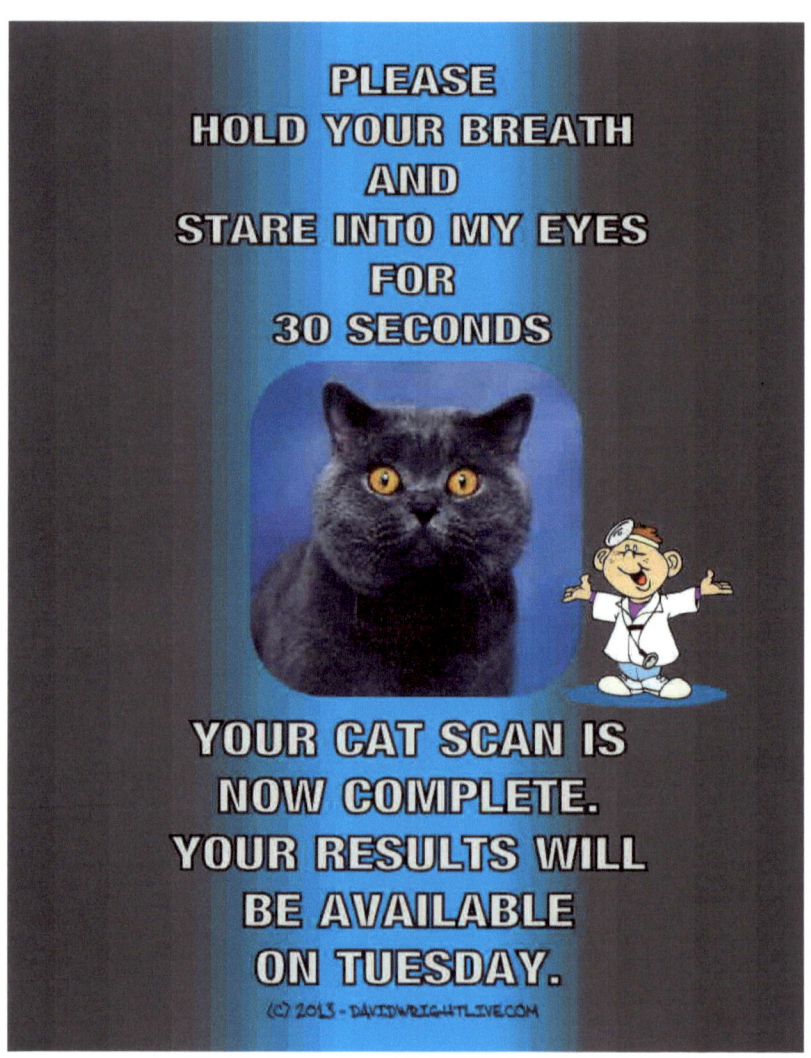

23ᴿᴰ PSALM IN PRAYER
AT THE CAT SCAN

The Lord is my shepherd, I shall not want;
<YOU MIGHT NOT WANT IT – BUT, YOUR DOCTOR DOES!>
He maketh me lie down in green pastures.
<OR - ON A TABLE FOR A CAT SCAN>
He leadeth me beside still waters;
<YES – YOU HAVE TO PEE, FIRST>
He restoreth my soul.
<HE EVEN HAS OTHERS ADDING THEIR STUFF
DIRECTLY THROUGH AN I.V.>
He leads me in paths of righteousness for his name's sake.
<AND, YOU WILL BE YELLING HIS NAME OUT LOUD
WHEN THE MEDS GO INTO YOUR VEINS –
SOMETHING LIKE THIS: "OH, GOD – OH, JESUS!">
Tho' I walk through the valley of the shadow of death,
I shall fear no evil;
<UNLESS THE OPERATOR HAS HAD A HISTORY OF
VISITING YOUR OLD BUSINESS - "LIQUOR 'R' US">
for thou art with me;
<HE IS RIGHT THERE WITH YOU - GUARANTEED>
thy rod and thy staff,
<YES, YOU WILL BE BEATEN SOUNDLY WITH
A ROD BY THE STAFF IF YOU DON'T COMPLY...>
they comfort me.
<...BUT, WILL BE NICE OTHERWISE.>
Thou preparest a table before me in
the presence of my enemies;
<OK – LAY DOWN ON THE TABLE, AND GET IT OVER WITH -
THE STAFF IS SEARCHING FOR THEM!>
thou anointest my head with oil,
<PUT THE TOWEL OVER YOUR FACE AS YOU SLIDE IN>
my cup overflows.
<OOOPS– I GUESS THE I.V. HAS SIDE EFFECTS, HUH?>
Surely, goodness and mercy shall follow me
all the days of my life;
<IT WILL – BUT, DON'T CALL ME SHIRLEY!>
and I shall dwell in the house of the Lord forever.
<NOT AS SOON YOU THINK –
THAT'S WHY YOU ARE GETTING THIS DONE NOW!>
AMEN.

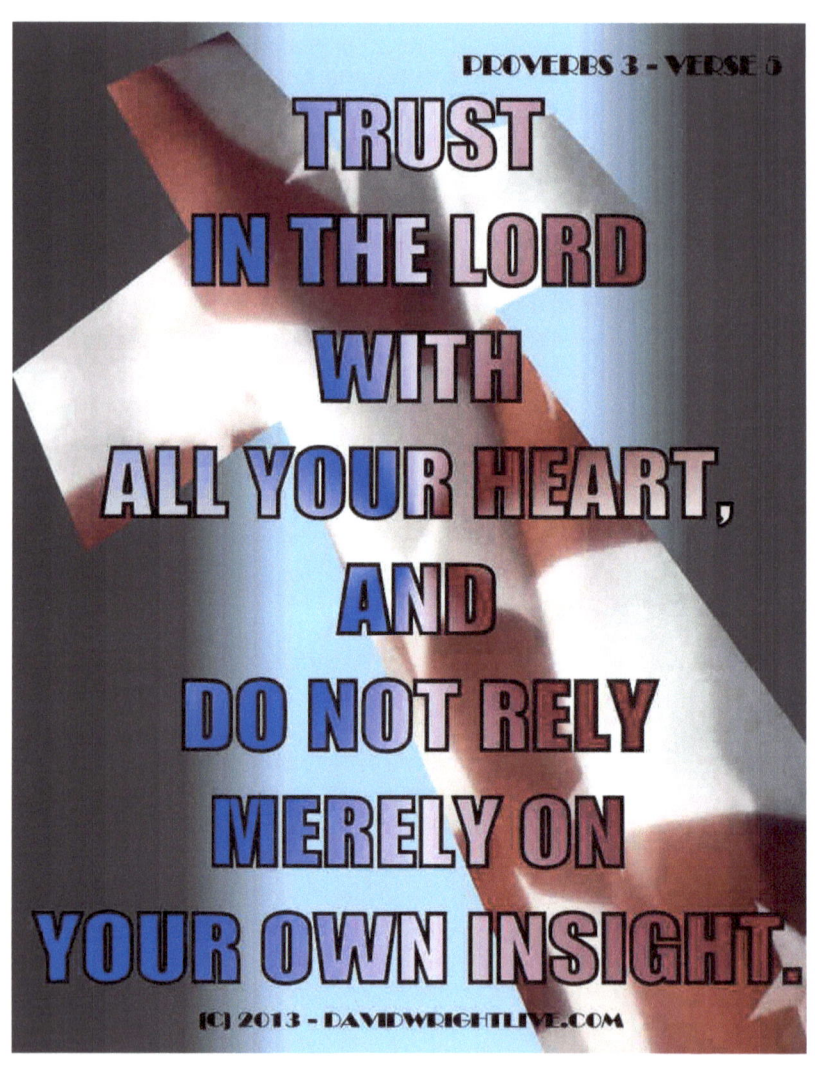

IT IS TIME TO
LET GO AND LET GOD

YEAR ONE

I affirm today, that by holding onto
negative expectations or doubt,
I will remove myself from the possibilities of
positive change, or, new and wondrous joy,
which is given abundantly by my God Within.
Conversely, I will affirm today, that by
expecting only the best, and most positive outcome,
and then making room for it within my heart
as a permanent part of my life, my
God Within will provide the Divine Wisdom I need.
Understanding this fundamental truth,
in the sacred silence of meditation and prayer,
I am enabled to express my innermost concerns,
and release them to God Himself,
for Him to handle them on my behalf.
By setting aside an uninterruptable time of
sacred meditative silence, I create the vaccuum
into which goodness and mercy comes rushing to
provide a greater understanding of my circumstances.
By releasing worries and fear to God,
I never need to take them back.
I have let them go, and am placing my trust
faithfully and completley in God to
create a brand new life for me.
As I read today, in
Proverbs 3, Verse 5,

*"TRUST IN THE LORD WITH ALL YOUR HEART
AND DO NOT RELY MERELY ON
YOUR OWN INSIGHT."*

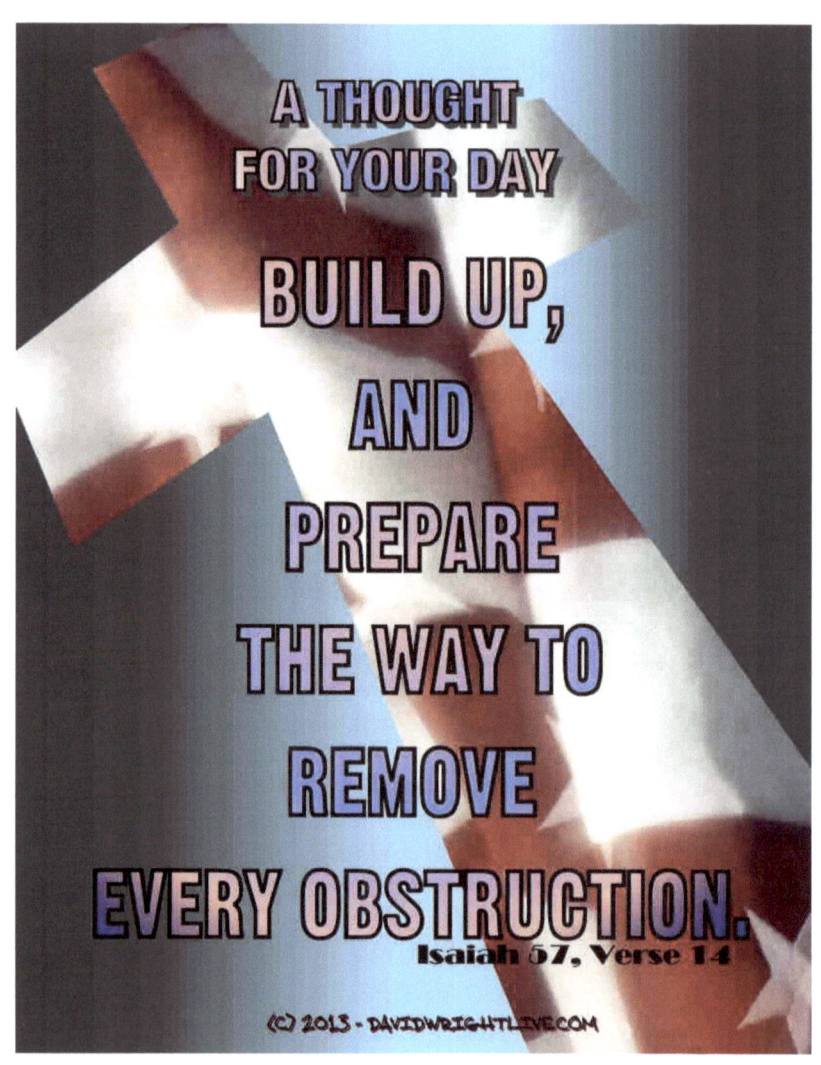

IT IS TIME TO ## *LET GO AND LET GOD*

YEAR TWO

Having reached a crossroads in the plan God has given me for
good, I am once again, at another point of welcomed refuge.
In the sacred silence of meditation and prayer,
I am enabled spiritually to pause while
reviewing and releasing my concerns.
A sense of calm washes over me, much as reaching an oasis
on a seemingly endless journey through a desert with no
recognizable landmarks.
As I pause, I listen to the unmistakable Inner Voice, and to the
options placed before me, with unshakable faith, taking
the path that I now know will lead me to the greatest good.
Today, as I let go, and let God guide me,
I will glance backward to take a last look at the place
from which I came, and will now set out once again
in a new direction with the knowledge that
He walks beside me through the most perfect
yet traversable storm.
Enfolded in the arms of God, and knowing that He loves me,
I look ahead without fear or trepidation, and
resume my life's journey, realizing that I am wearing a
newly polished set of boots to take me there.
This morning, as I read in Isaiah 57, Verse 14,
I will begin this journey knowing I should

*"BUILD UP, AND PREPARE THE WAY TO
REMOVE EVERY OBSTRUCTION."*

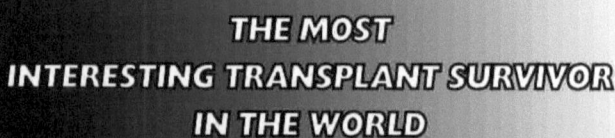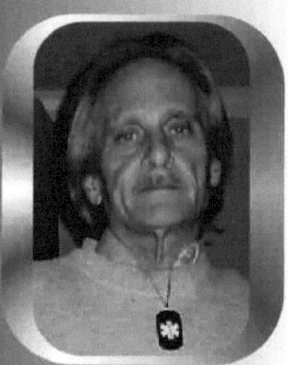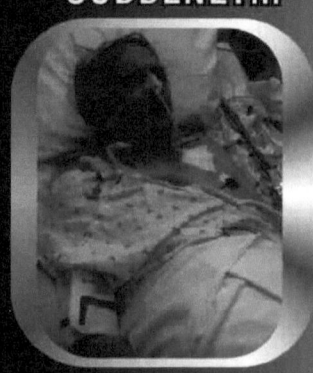

WITH GOD, ANYTHING IS POSSIBLE

YEAR THREE

As I awaken this morning, after listening to
my Inner Voice and expressing the
WILLINGNESS TO LET GO and LET GOD,
and accepting the abundance of blessings
that I am about to receive, I have learned that
whatever I can conceive and believe, I can achieve.
In the sacred silence of meditation and prayer,
I willingly open my heart and mind to the
Divine Instruction He gives in the loving creation
of a personal endowment of well being.
Today, I will allow His Presence to
beome my Guiding Light.
With my faith, and His Divine Guidance,
I can achieve all that I can now believe about
all that is presented to me on my behalf
knowing it is a gift of Divine Wisdom.
Turning to scripture, I read
Ephesians 3, Verse 20, which says,

*"NOW TO HIM WHO BY THE
POWER AT WORK WITHIN US
IS ABLE TO ACCOMPLISH ABUNDANTLY
FAR MORE THAN WE CAN ASK OR IMAGINE
IS GLORY."*

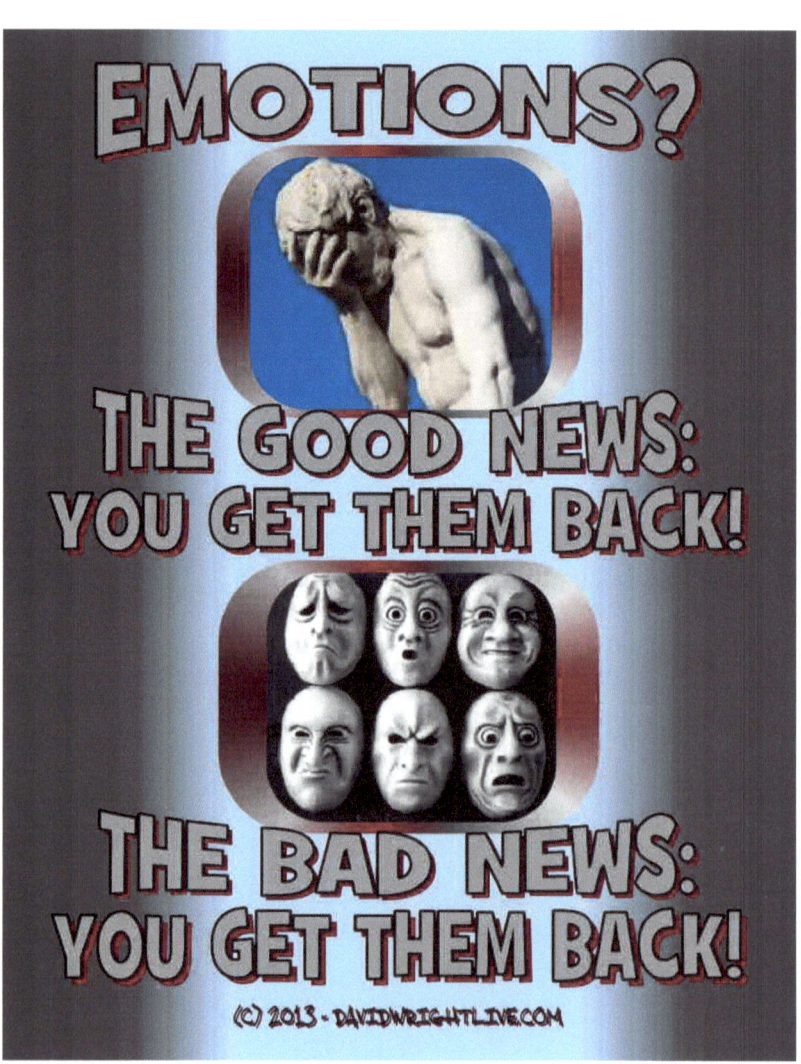

LET GO AND LET GOD
IN QUIET AFFIRMATION

YEAR FOUR

As I awaken this morning,
I have become more enthusiastic than ever
about life and the good flowing inward that is
ultimately awaiting me today.
Opening my eyes, I am ready to receive that
which I need to know, and what the next step
on my journey will be.
Having released any thought of physical or
emotional pain from past events and circumstances,
I am clearing the way for a successful
healing transformation to begin.
Focusing on the presence of my God Within,
once again,
I quietly affirm:
I LET GO and LET GOD.
I am no longer being burdened with trying to "fix" my life.
I realize, with a new clarity, what I can do to
enhance my life,
and am willing to become a partner in the
co-operative success of this incredible upcoming adventure.
As I let go and let God,
I immediately feel at peace with myself.
God's guidance brings me greater peace, broader perspectives,
clarity, and a truer understanding of
how we can all work together, and achieve success.
Today, in Psalm 16, Verse 11, I read,

"YOU SHOW ME THE PATH OF LIFE.
IN YOUR PRESENCE THERE IS
FULLNESS OF JOY."

THE MOST INTERESTING TRANSPLANT SURVIVOR IN THE WORLD

WE CANNOT SOLVE OUR PROBLEMS WITH THE SAME THINKING WE USED WHEN WE CREATED THEM.

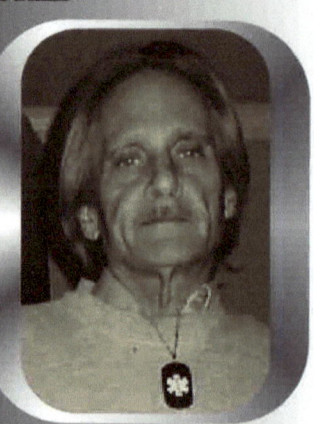

IT'S NOT THAT I'M SO SMART, IT'S JUST THAT I AM WILLING TO STAY WITH PROBLEMS LONGER.

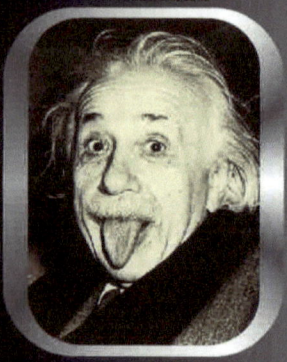

KEEP BREATHING, MY FRIEND!

(C) 2013 - DAVIDWRIGHTLIVE.COM

LET GO AND LET GOD
PATIENTLY

YEAR FIVE

As I awaken this morning, and begin to listen to
my Inner Voice, I am not just patiently waiting,
but realize that all around me,
all with whom I come into contact,
have been placed on an intersecting path with me
where we will come together to reach the solutions
most necessary for my health and well being.
Releasing any negative energy within, and
letting God take it upon His Shoulders to bear,
I can focus on the further development of patience
as I observe all the good that is
now happening on my behalf.
By releasing the negative energy surrounding me,
I create a vaccuum within to patiently await
drawing forth the positive energy of all of those
who are here with me on this journey.
Joyfully, I willingly accept and acknowledge the
best options and considerations at this time.
By proactively responding to Spirit within me,
I no longer react with haste or without thought.
Through His Divine Comfort, I relax, and feel at ease
knowing that all is being done in God's perfect timing.
As I read in James 5, Verse 7,

"BE PATIENT, THEREFORE BELOVED,
UNTIL THE COMING OF THE LORD."

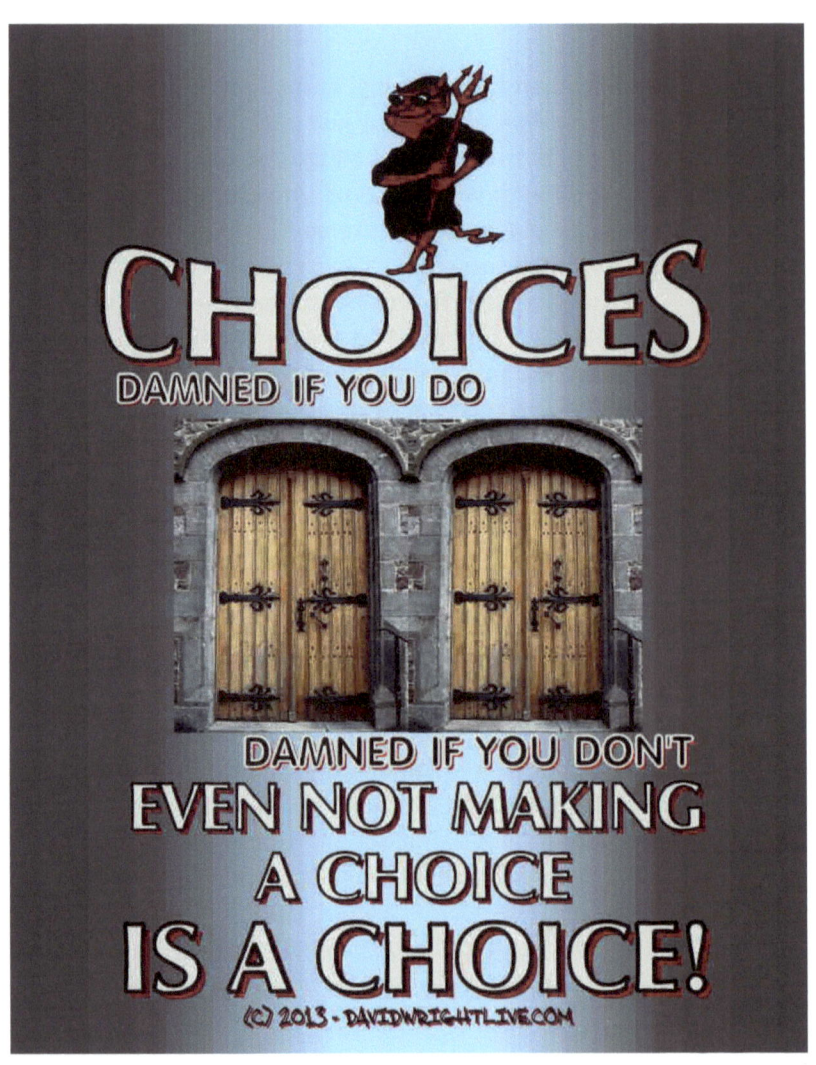

LET GO AND LET GOD
TRUST THE CHOICES

YEAR SIX

As I awaken this morning, I realize when listening
to my Inner Voice, that within God's Plan for me,
I have been given an abundance of positive choices
that are designed to lead to positive outcomes.
Stepping outside that which was comfortable
so long ago before this path was taken,
I willingly have new experiences which
make my joyful spirit soar.
I will make conscious choices with complete
faith and trust in my God Within.
I willingly choose to let go of the
fear of the unknown
as I soar with exhilaration and excitement
and enjoy taking each new step along the way.
I choose to recognize that God is within me,
and I am always using His Divine Wisdom.
I feel liberated, and open myself to
God's perfect
expresssion from within me.
Knowing all is well, I choose not to worry about
potential outcomes, as I know if God is for me,
who could possibly be against me?
Divinely Blessed by God
I am always
Guided and Protected.
My choice of scripture for the day is,
Isaiah 26, Verse 4,

"TRUST IN THE LORD FOREVER."

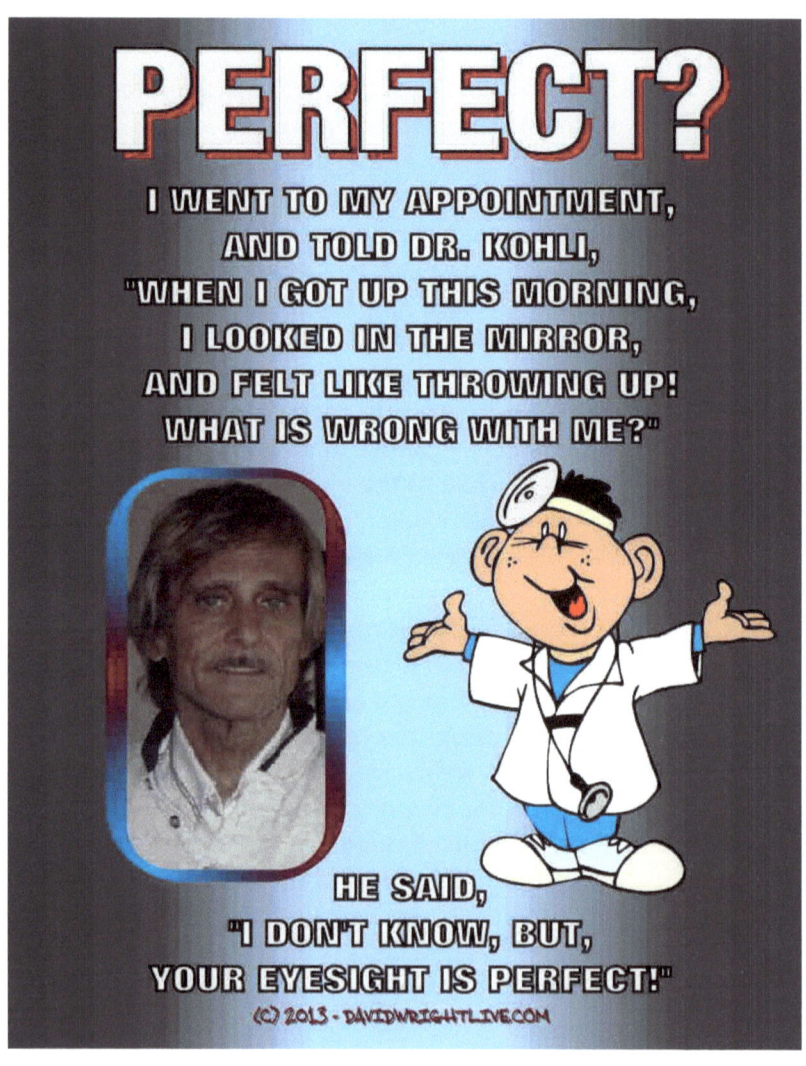

LET GO AND LET GOD
DO THE PREPARATION

YEAR SEVEN

As I awaken this morning, and am
listening to my Inner Voice,
I am, once again, preparing to take
yet another leap of faith into the unknown.
I will let go of all personal expectations, and
let God reveal His Infinite Possibilities to me.
Revealing my Highest Good within the Divine Order
he has created, my faith assures me that
WITH GOD ALL THINGS ARE POSSIBLE.
While the achievement of healthful success results
requires following a series of well-executed steps,
if I should stumble along the way,
I won't give up on Him, on myself, or on
the team who has gathered forces to help me succeed.
Having my God Within as a constant companion in life,
I turn to Him whenever I may reach a new obstacle,
and together, in the sacred silence of
meditation and prayer, we will find the right direction.
As my God Within guides me to the fulfillment of
my Highest Good, I receive blessing after blessing.
Whenever I let go, and let God,
I learn from each new experience.
Today will be a joyful day of new experiences.
As I read in Psalm 56, Verses 10 and 11,

"IN GOD, WHOSE WORD I PRAISE...
IN GOD I TRUST; I AM UNAFRAID."

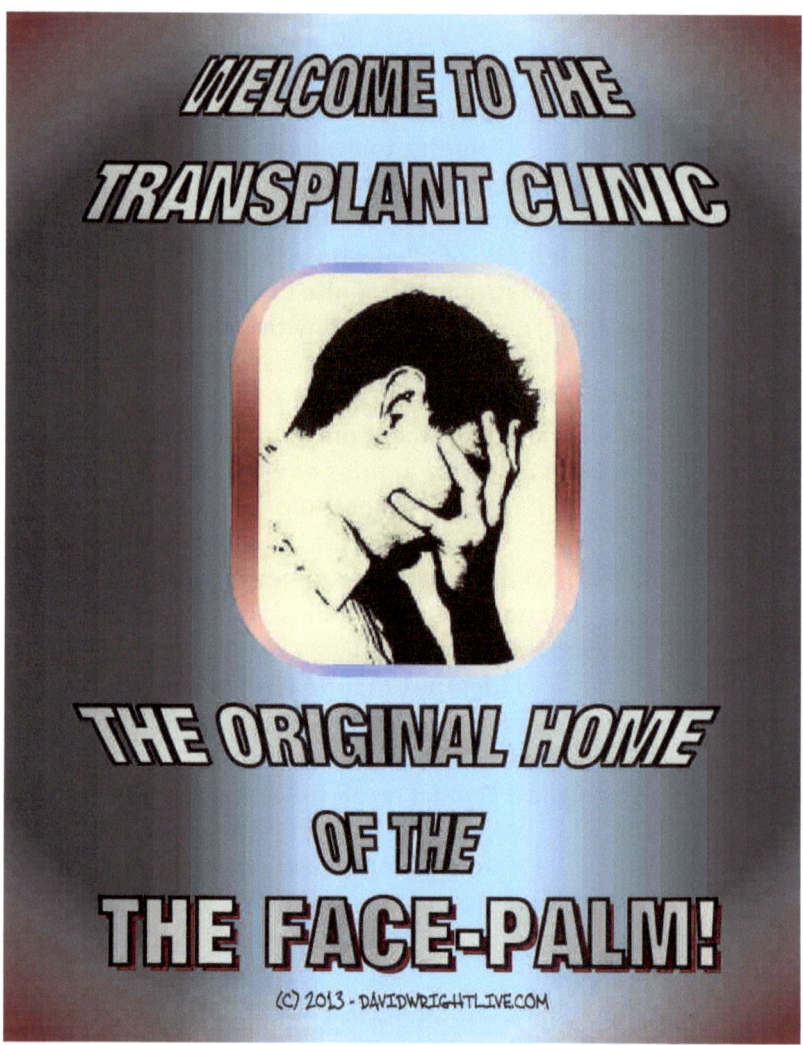

LET GO, AND LET GOD
HANDLE THE CONTROLS

YEAR EIGHT

As I awaken this morning,
feeling unusally at odds with my Inner Voice,
affirming a strong desire to develop and maintain
more control over this upcoming event in my life,
I am learning that my inflexibility may actually
become a blockage to the Divine Wisdom
my God Within is there to provide.
As a reminder of enabling myself to feel
more at peace, I will step back, take a time out,
and deeply breathe in His Love from all around me.
I willingly place my trust, once again,
in the knowledge that I am on His Path, and that each
member of my personal support team is there to
follow the plan God has for them to provide for me.
I can free myself from control issues by
allowing the situation to unfold around me as
a spectator would watch a sporting match in a stadium.
I will trust His Divine Wisdom to guide my thoughts,
and those of my team, in words, deeds and actions.
I willingly accept this freedom and peace.
As I read this morning in Proverbs 16, Verse 9,

*"THE HUMAN MIND PLANS THE WAY,
BUT, THE LORD DIRECTS THE STEPS."*

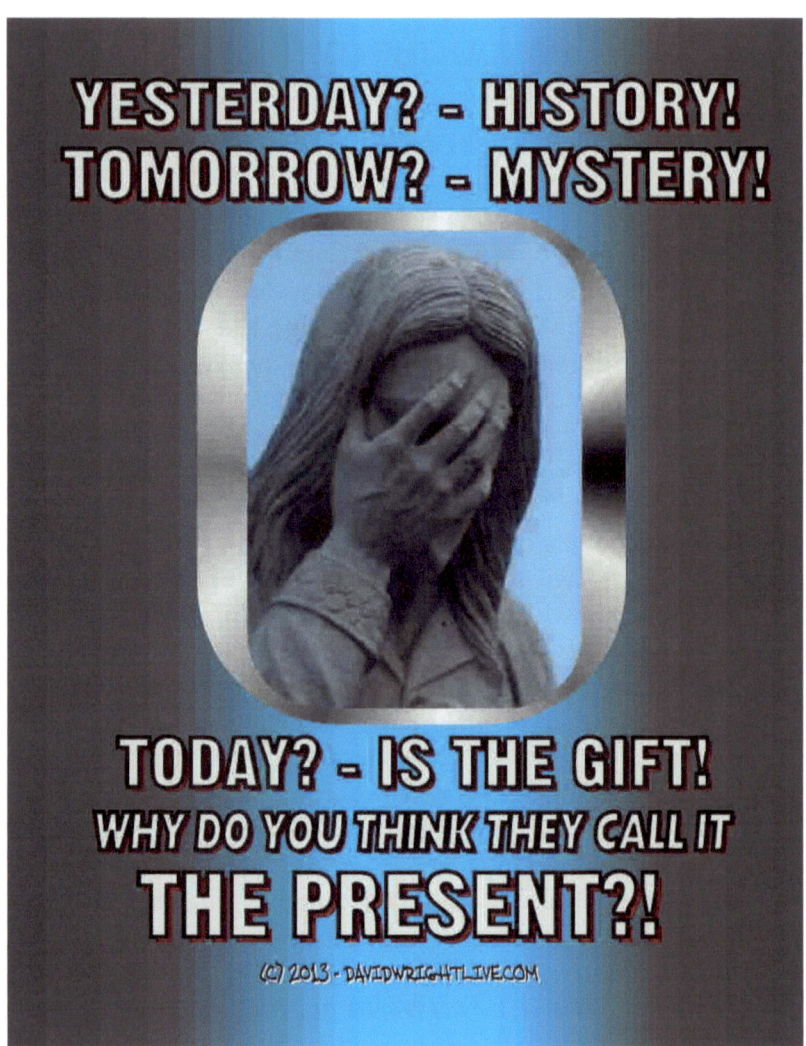

EXAMINING THE PRECIOUS PRESENT

YEAR NINE

As I awaken this morning, I willingly listen
intently to the Inner Voice for the Divine Wisdom
which will show me, once again,
how to live this, and every subsequent day
of those with which I will be blessed,
one precious moment at a time.
Feeling at ease in this moment, in whatever form
it must take, I realize that
this is the day the Lord has made, and
I will now rejoice and be glad in it.
Unable to change that which is past, I will focus
on living on this planet today under the weight
of my circumstances, as God has presented them
to me within the plan He has for me –
a plan for good – always.
I am grateful for each moment, and each opportunity
for the recognition of the fulfillment of His promises.
As I am sharing the current coursing of my life with those
around me, those who care deeply for me, who
wish nothing but the best of every eventual outcome,
I am grateful that this is yet another day
for me to live life well.
This morning, in Matthew 6 , Verse 11, I read,

"GIVE US THIS DAY, OUR DAILY BREAD."

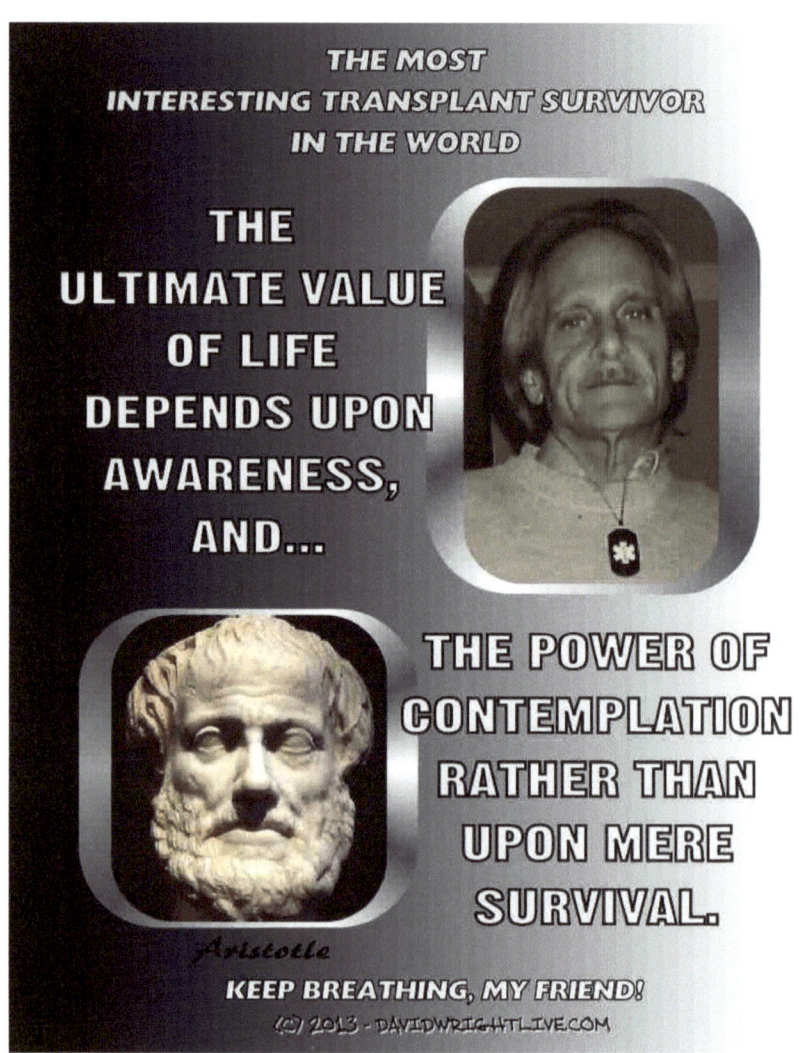

RECOGNIZING
THE VALUE OF LIFE

YEAR TEN

As I awaken this morning, once again, and
listen enthusiastically to my Inner Voice,
in the sacred silence of meditation and prayer,
I recognize the value of life in all of its forms.
Every moment in the precious present, and in the
forseeable future, is of incredible value as I travel
the path that God has planned uniquely for me.
The progress I have made, and will make,
is measured now with daily milestones.
Every step and breath I take, is
ANOTHER MIRACLE OF MY CREATOR.
Every new experience and realization is
yet another movement forward in my
personal spiritual growth and development.
Traveling this path, with God by my side,
I willingly become more and more aware of my
Divine Guidance, personal power and passion for life.
Each day, one moment at a time, I am brought closer
to understanding the intentions of my God Within,
and the hurdles He has chosen for me to face.
On what is becoming a sacred personal journey,
my God Within provides the safety and comfort I need.
As I read in Timothy 4, Verse 15,

*"PUT THESE THINGS INTO PRACTICE,
AND DEVOTE YOURSELF TO THEM,
SO THAT ALL MAY SEE YOUR PROGRESS."*

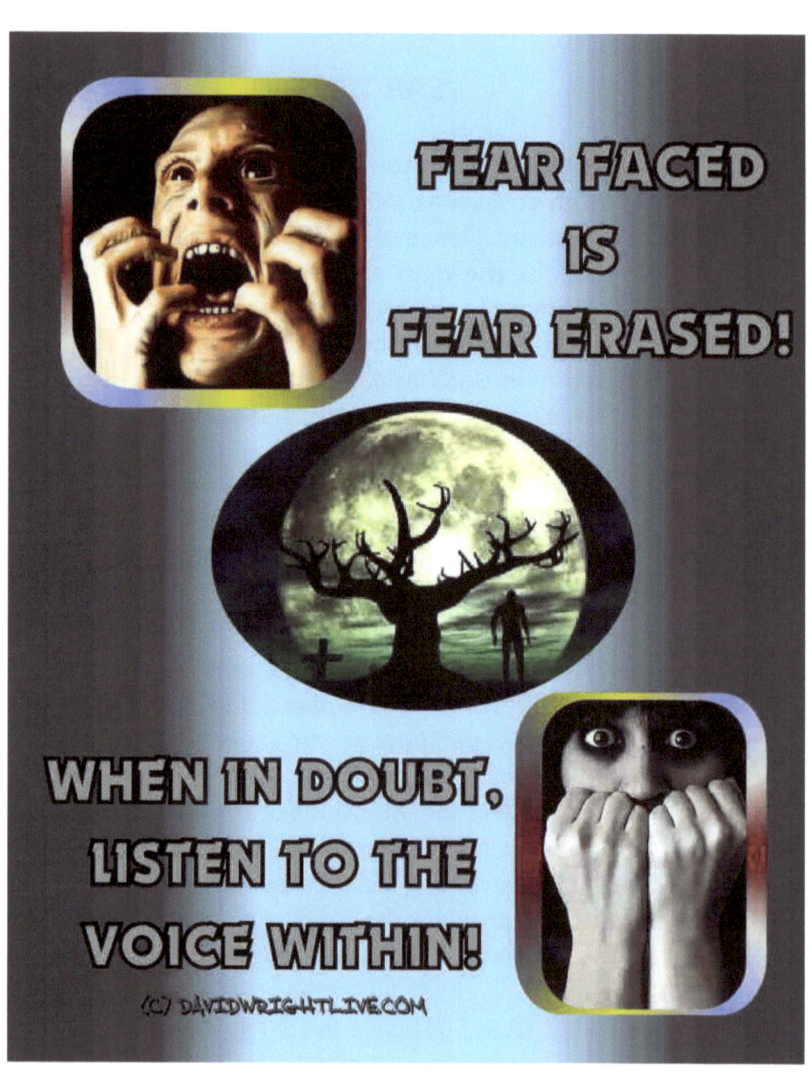

*PROVIDED WITH
A WELLNESS INFUSION*

YEAR ELEVEN

As I awaken this morning, I listen as my Inner Voice
provides the details of an upcoming wellness infusion.
Infused daily with the life giving energy provided by
my God Within, I am becoming one with Spirit,
and the life force itself of God at work.
In the sacred silence of meditation and prayer,
I visualize how to harness the energy from
all of those around me, learn about it, and
focus it in the areas that need it most.
Undaunted, I am no longer defined by a diagnosis,
as the healing light of God Within is infusing
every cell and every organ, new or old,
throughout my body.
Willingly, I affirm that I am completely prepared
to deny admittance to anything that might stand
in the way of the acceptance of healing light
entering and doing its work within me.
I only need ask now for the complete awareness of
those around me to continue to provide prayer,
acceptance, and support of the healing power we
mutually bring forth in the spirit of love.
As I read this morning in Luke, Verse 19,

*"ALL IN THE CROWD WERE TRYING TO TOUCH HIM,
FOR POWER CAME OUT FROM HIM
AND HEALED ALL OF THEM."*

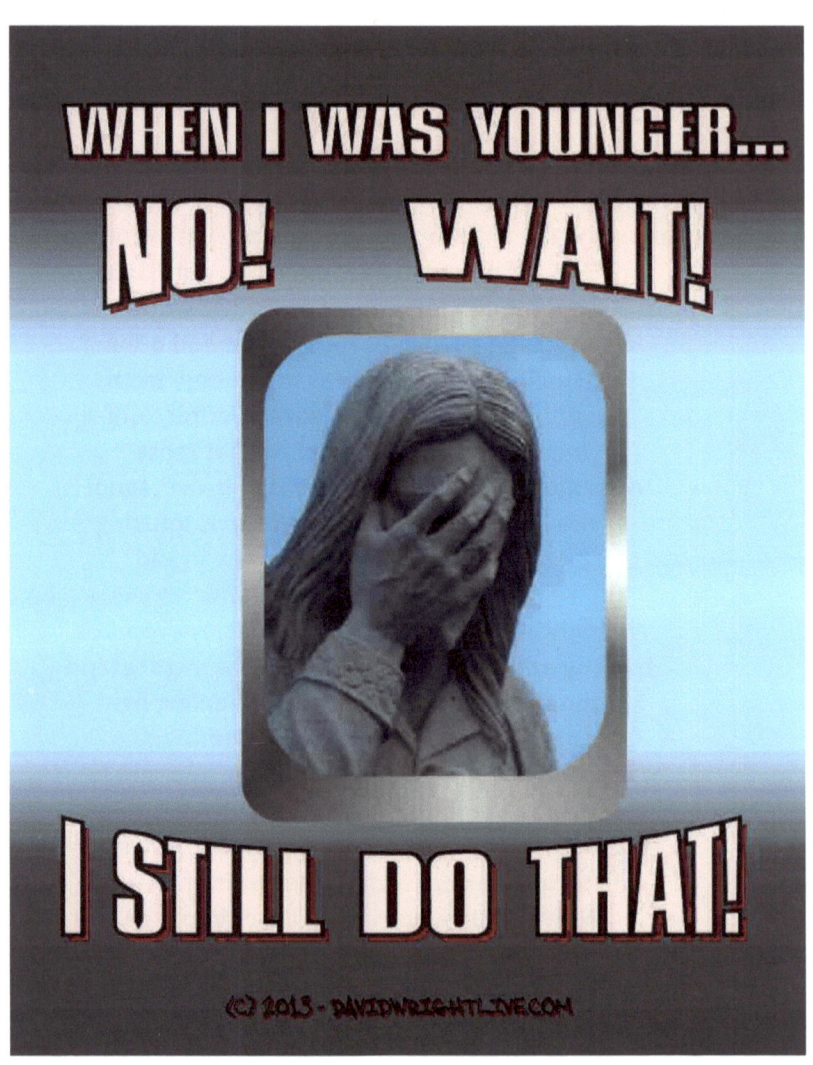

GRATITUDE
IN HARMONY

YEAR TWELVE

As I awaken this morning, and follow the direction of
my Inner Voice, gratefully, I will take the time to work with
family, friends, co-workers, and the instrumental support
providers so involved in my personal transformation, to
create a new level of harmony at every point in our lives
which will enable us to develop and enjoy all of these
new and wondrous moments of this entire experience.
Recognizing that each of us is a magnificent creation of God,
and each of us is one with God, I will demonstrate
my trust in the power and presence I have been given to
connect with them all to multiply our mutual happiness.
I will be eternally grateful for the
*SPIRITUAL, PHYSICAL, MENTAL
and EMOTIONAL ABILITIES*
with which I have been blessed that create
the celebration of shared efforts on this journey as we
find the willingness to search for a successful outcome.
In this quest, we are truly becoming one with God.
Releasing stress, letting go, and letting God,
I affirm that He is, indeed, working through me
to create the highest and greatest good.
As I read this morning in John 14, Verse 10,

*"THE FATHER WHO DWELLS IN ME
DOES HIS WORKS."*

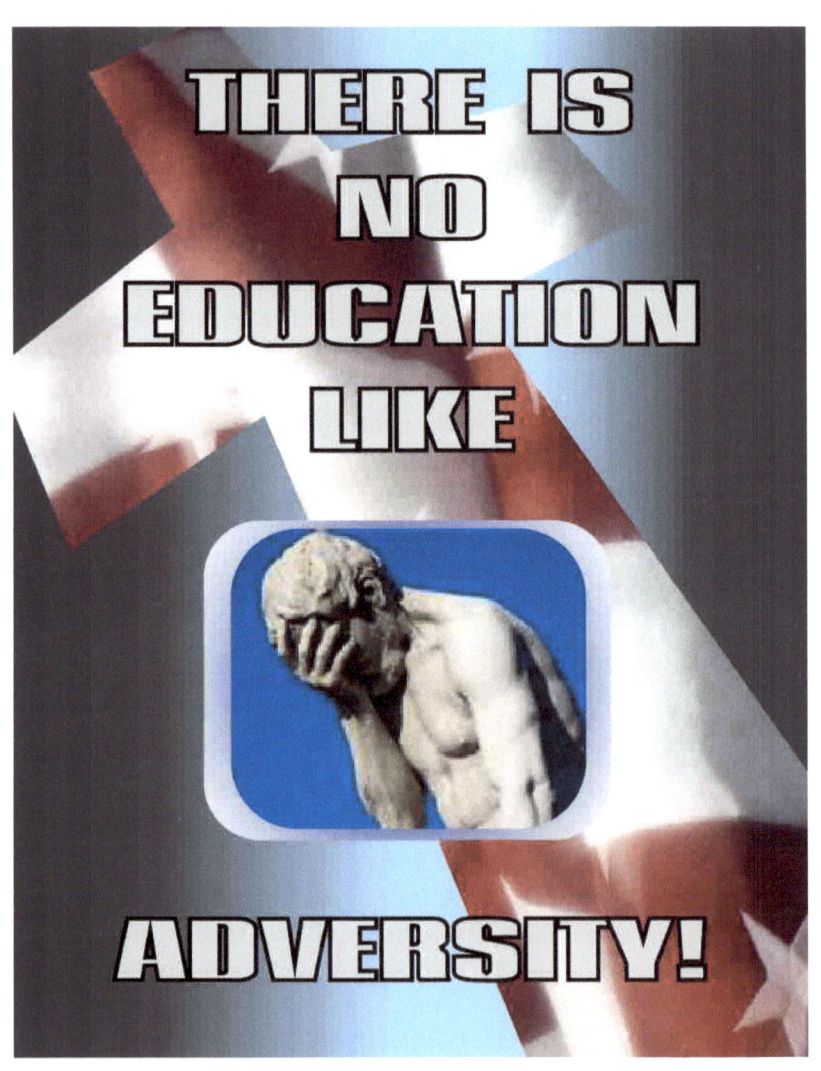

STRENGTH THROUGH FAITH

YEAR THIRTEEN

After awakening this morning, and spending
the time in the sacred silence of meditation and prayer,
gratefully, I realize while listening to my Inner Voice
that it is this time in which my spirit takes wing, and soars.
Today, I affirm that my God Within is my spiritual strength.
My faith is the power behind the ever-unfolding plan that
God has provided in such a perfect manner for my life.
My spiritual faith is now lifting me up every day as
my mind and body feel the wholeness of my God Within.
I am inspired to reach beyond that which I may have
considered as limitations, and will continue to aspire
to the most Divine Potential provided to me.
Establishing a firm conviction of belief in my Inner Voice
creates all that I need for this new beginning.
Letting go of fears and limitations, I will soar like an eagle
while continually applying the strength and ability
with which I have been so richly blessed.
As I place my faith in God,
my spirit soars to incredible new heights.
As I read in Psalm 84, Verse 5,

**"HAPPY ARE THOSE
WHOSE STRENGTH IS IN YOU."**

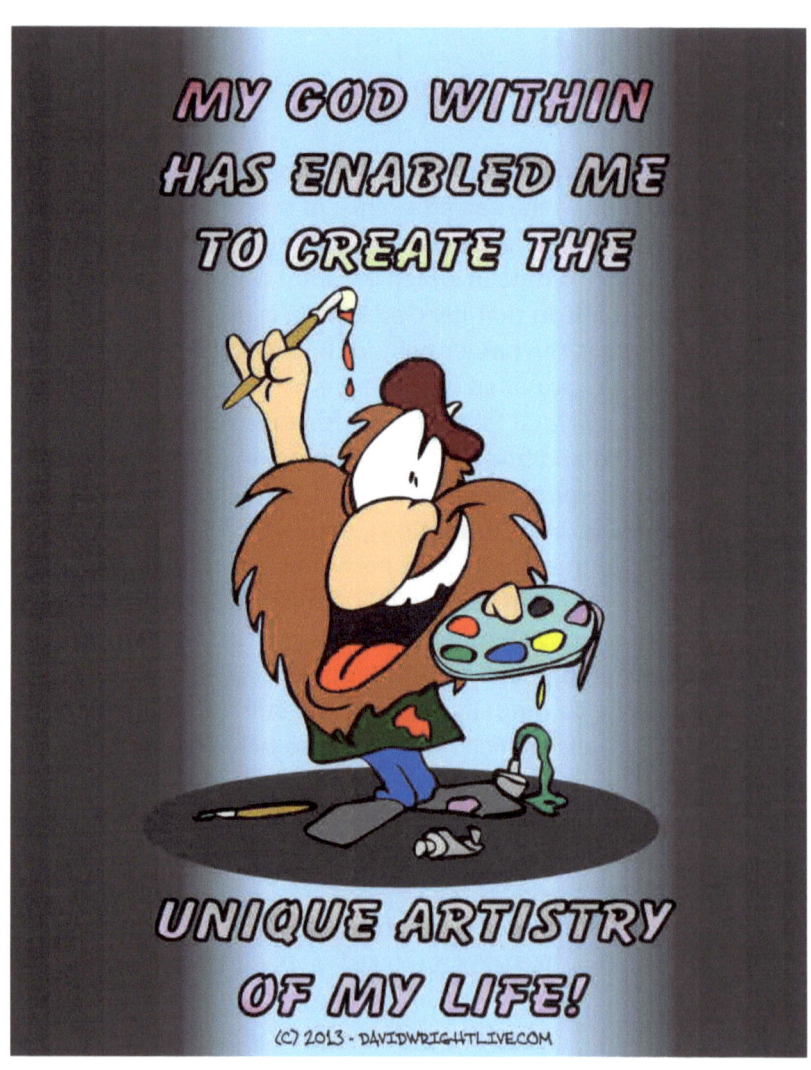

I HAVE BECOME THE ARTIST OF MY LIFE

YEAR FOURTEEN

As I awaken this morning, and listen closely
to my Inner Voice, I willingly acknowledge
my gratitdue to my God Within
for creating and providing the canvas on which
I am enabled to create the artistry of my unique life.
Everyone I meet and welcome into my life
along the way adds a new and even richer dimension
now as they contribute to the evolving masterpiece of
LIGHT, COLOR and CONTRAST
which I personally enjoy every day of my life.
I acknowledge my gratitude to my God Within as
I have learned to live a life filled with love.
My thoughts and feelings are now, as they always
have been, a creation of my lifetime of experience.
Breathing in deeply, I willingly acknowledge
the never-ending inflow of Divine Knowledge
with which I have become blessed.
Today, I will acknowledge my gratitude
with the words and actions that have become
so uniquely mine.
As I read in John 2, Verse 10,

*"WHO-SO-EVER LOVES, LIVES IN THE LIGHT,
AND IN SUCH A PERSON
THERE IS NO CAUSE FOR STUMBLING."*

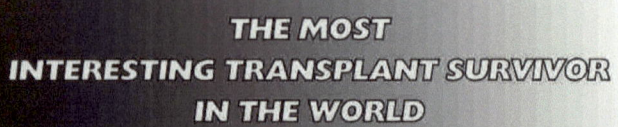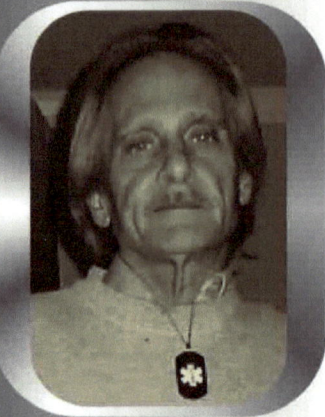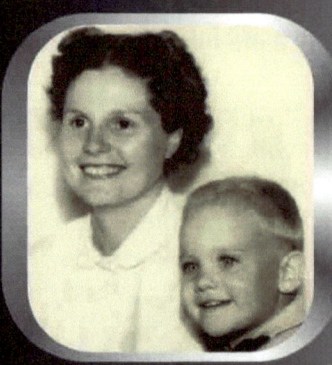

THE ATTITUDE IS ALWAYS GRATITUDE

YEAR FIFTEEN

I could not be more grateful to my God Within
For being born of parents like mine.
Did you have parents who loved and cared about
The family, while making each day divine?
Did they take the time to teach what's important,
And never found the time to whine?
Yes, I have learned to be grateful for my God Within.

Are you grateful to your God Within today,
For learning graciously to accept mistakes?
Do you celebrate each day as you learn once again,
The difference that faith always makes?
Finding health in body, and in relationships,
Are yours, when willing to do what it takes.
Yes, I have learned to be grateful for my God Within.

You can put the keys to happiness in your pocket.
It's time now to stop giving them away.
The Inner Voice of my God Within answers
My prayers, and out loud, you will hear me say,
He gives me the strength and guidance that I need
On this, and on every single day.
Yes, I have learned to be grateful for my God Within.

I have been blessed with the plan He has given me,
It is unique, just like the one he has given to you.
As I take it step by step on this arduous journey,
I'm not the first, and believe me, neither are you.
Walking through the Valley of the Shadow of Death
I'll be leaving a footprint, or two.
*Yes, I have learned to be grateful for my God Within,
...for He is always walking there with me.*

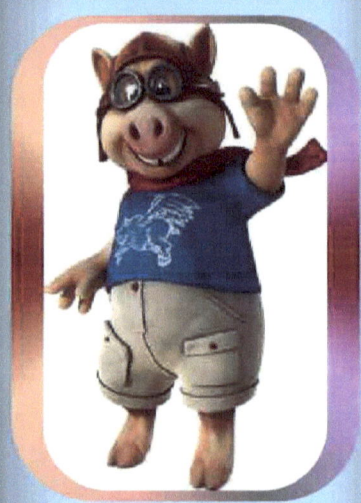

THE COMFORT OF FREEDOM

YEAR SIXTEEN

As I awaken this morning, free and unlimited,
listening to my Inner Voice, I rest assured in
the steadfast
LOVE of my GOD WITHIN.
So much more than a mere state of being,
freedom is a complete state of mind.
By opening my heart and mind to my God Within,
I am strengthened and comforted by being given
His Divine Guidance which will release me
from the chains of limitation in my own thinking.
I have been released from the limitations
imposed by others as well.
My Inner Voice will continually guide me
through any experience bravely and courageously.
I willingly begin this and every day to follow
knowing I am not alone and always in
His Divine and Loving Care.
Living within this state of freedom, and
feeling wrapped in a comforting blanket of
GOD's LOVE,
I willingly begin my journey again today,
enthusiastically, with a
free spirit and a joyful heart.
As I read in Psalm 119, Verse 76,

"LET YOUR STEADFAST LOVE BECOME MY COMFORT ACCORDING TO YOUR PROMISE TO YOUR SERVANT."

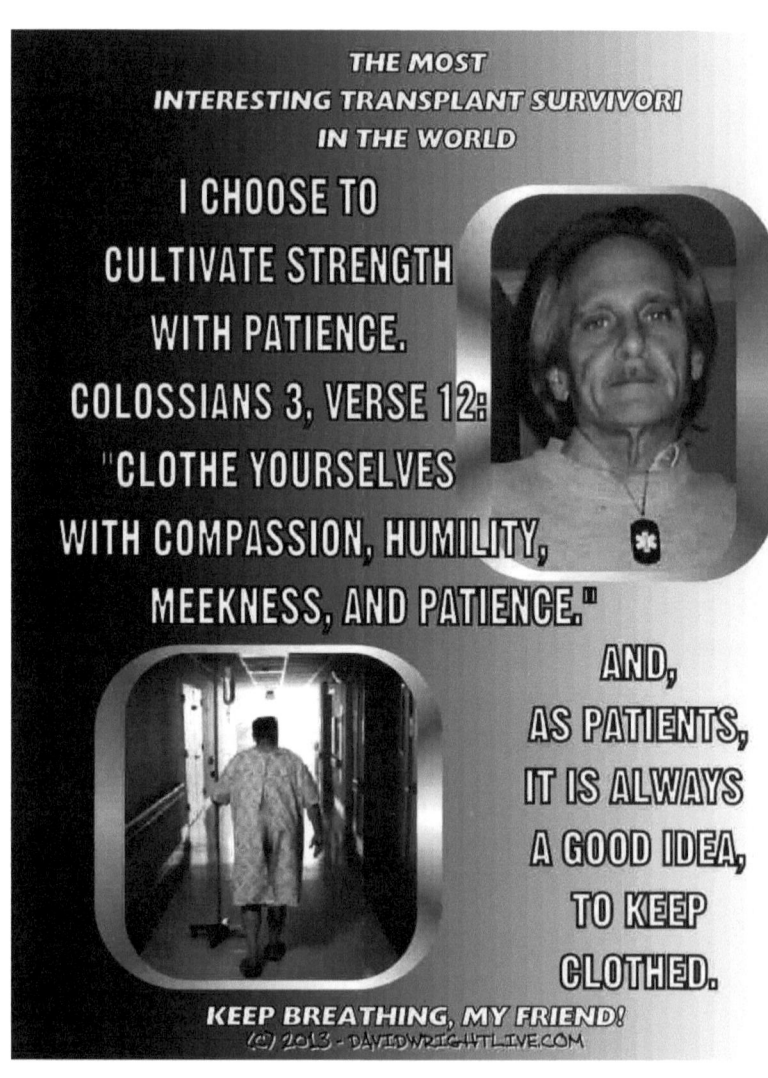

A CHOICE OF PATIENCE

YEAR SEVENTEEN

As I awaken this morning, I choose to listen to
my Inner Voice, acknowledging that I am always
given the opportunity to use Divine Knowledge.
Having learned through faith over many years
that all good things happen in God's Perfect Timing,
once again today, I will choose to cultivate ever
more strength with patience.
In the sacred silence of meditation and prayer
I willingly affirm that,
"There is a time for every purpose under heaven."
While waiting patiently in silent prayer,
With steadfast resolve, I will approach the tasks at hand
with conversation that is filled purposely with
kindness and understanding for others,
with a patient heart and mind, just as it has been
shown to me time and time again over this long
and difficult journey.
In building my resolve, in renewing my faith,
as I have so many times before, I find it helpful
again today, to read Colossians 3, Verse 12,

**"CLOTHE YOURSELVES WITH
COMPASSION, HUMILITY,
MEEKNESS AND PATIENCE."**

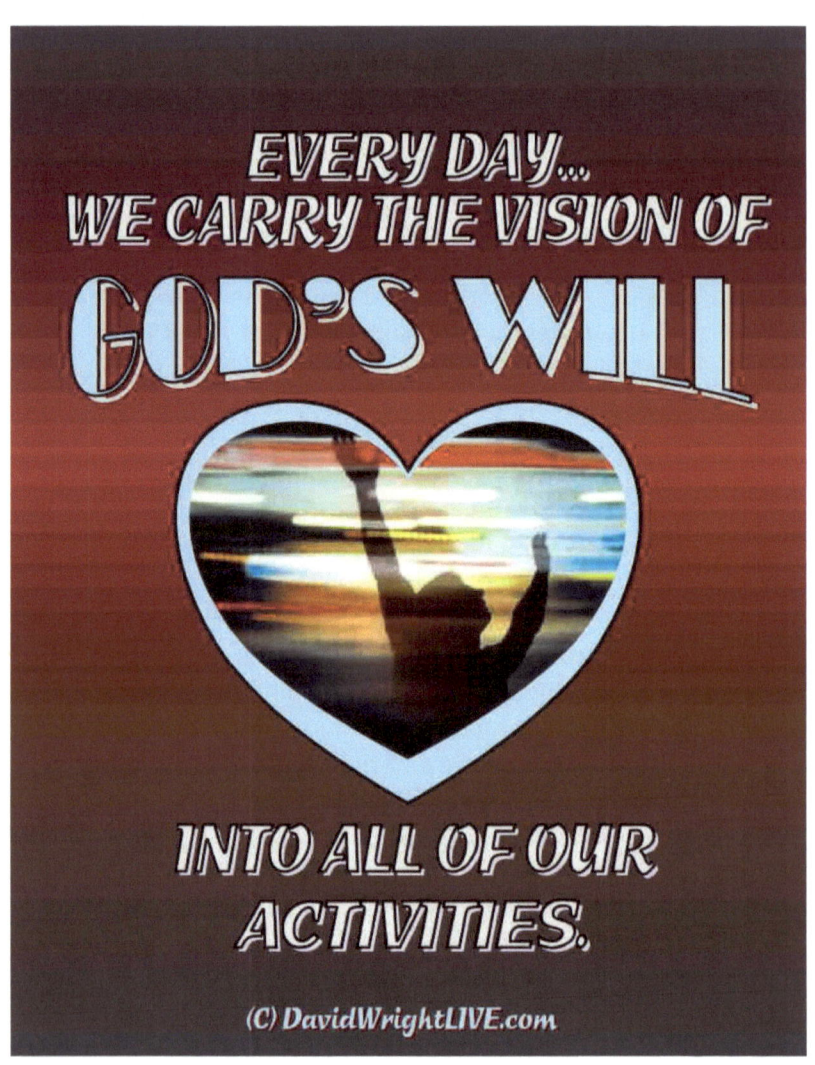

DIVINE WISDOM LEADS TO
THE RIGHT OUTCOME

YEAR EIGHTEEN

As I awaken this morning, I listen to the Inner Voice, and
am finding myself, over and over, being led to
THE RIGHT OUTCOME IN EVERY SITUATION.
Becoming open to the Divine Wisdom of my God Within
before starting a new project, or a new relationship,
I am finding more and more goals to pursue, and
everything goes smoothly in anticipation of success.
In the sacred silence of meditation and prayer,
I listen to a variety of considerations for reaching a solution,
and find a blessing when I set aside the selfish need
of always having my own way.
By releasing the all too human tendency to control,
I have learned to *LET GO, and LET GOD,*
and to faithfully follow Divine Wisdom.
Every concern I have disappears, and everything falls
into its perfect place with perfect harmony.
The Light of God's Presence Within
will always light the way.
This morning, I read Psalm 143, Verse 10, which says,

"TEACH ME TO DO YOUR WILL, FOR YOU ARE MY GOD.
LET YOUR SPIRIT OF GOODNESS LEAD ME
ON A LEVEL PATH."

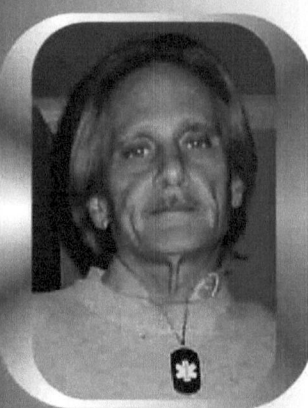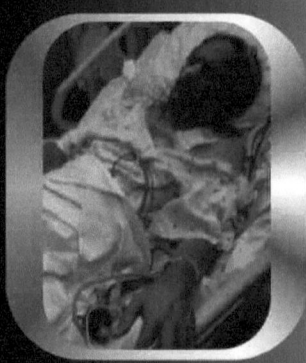

THE MIRACLE OF MY NEW LIFE

YEAR NINETEEN

As I awaken this morning, I am reminded by my
Inner Voice that the miracle of life exists within
the inner complexity and the external beauty of
the physical temple we call our body.
Each of us is blessed with cells, tissues and organs
constructed within
A FRAMEWORK OF DIVINE ENGINEERING.
Throughout the day, working tirelessly, our God Within
protects, repairs, and regenerates every physical aspect
of what we are currently using.
When another has no more need for their physical temple,
but has left behind that from which we can rebuild,
God is working the plan as the master renovator.
Blessed with the Divine Knowledge of those around me
who have followed their Inner Voice, I embrace the
deepest gratitude for the newest part of the
Divine Life I now share without ever knowing who
so graciously gave this gift to me.
I will become the radiant embodiment of strength
as I am embracing my new gift with gratitude
as all that flows within me now is vitality.
As I read this morning in Corinthians 6, Verse 19,

"DO YOU NOT KNOW THAT
YOUR BODY IS A TEMPLE OF
THE HOLY SPIRIT WITHIN,
AND YOU ARE NOT YOUR OWN?"

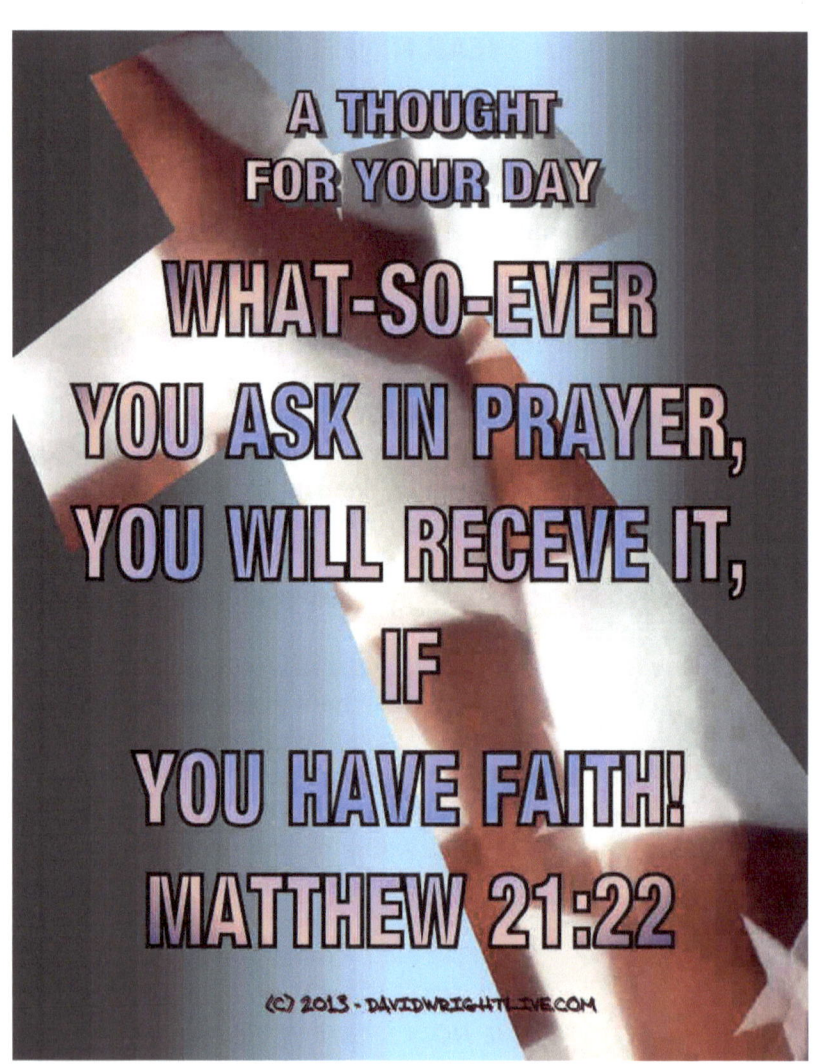

THE ULTIMATE GIFT
GRATITUDE

YEAR TWENTY

Awakening today, twenty years after it all began,
and just shortly after the one big expected step,
I realized that as I listened to the Inner Voice, and
began to open my heart and mind, I grew ever stronger,
and developed gratitude for what I have been given.
I am grateful, far more than I ever could have understood
without this experience, for having been given the
ultimate gift

- LIFE -

NOT ONCE, BUT TWICE.

Every day now is a perfect day as I spend it with the
people who matter most to me, my companion animals,
and well-wishers, always surrounded in love,
immersed in faith and joy, and continuing to learn
ever more about life, love, and laughter,
while reaching an even greater potential every day.
In the sacred silence of meditation and prayer,
I hear the Inner Voice, and always still pay
close attention.
I pray for those who are taking a similar journey,
and that they take the time to listen as well,
as the destination is not the reward.
It is the journey.
Joyfully, I live in gratitude – it's an attitude.

THANK YOU EVERYONE.
THANK YOU, GOD.

THE POWER OF PRAYER

Do you believe in the power of prayer?
My friend, now you know I do.
I let go of my problems, and gave them to God,
It was then that I wrote this to you.

I have learned that there are four ways
From which He'll choose to answer you.
I have learned all about the patience we need
While he is following through.

Sometimes, He gives us exactly what we want,
Overnight, or even today.
Then, there are times we have to wait much longer,
Months or years, not right away.

At times, we won't be given what we ask for,
Because we didn't know what was best.
Instead, it's what we really wanted or needed,
But, we had to understand the test.

Most times, we do not get what we wanted,
No matter how often we object or digress.
Rest assured though, what we will always be given
Is what He knows to be the very best.

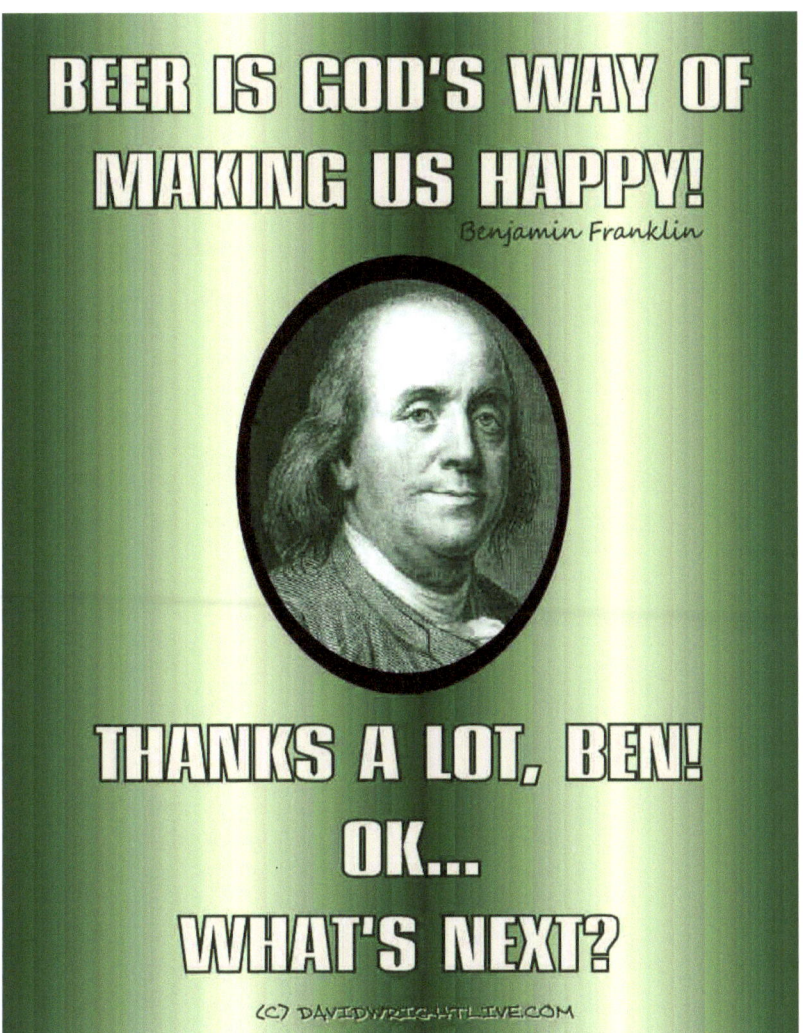

VISION

And God said,
Let there be Light.
And God saw the Light,
and that it was good;
and, He separated the
Light from the darkness.
Genesis 1:3,4

You are the
Light of the World.
A city on a hill
cannot be hidden.
Matthew 5:14

(C) 2013 - DAVIDWRIGHTLIVE.COM

WHAT'S NEXT?
VISION – MISSION
PHILOSOPHY - SYSTEMS

Having been given the gift of a new life, and having the benefit of lessons learned from the earlier one, we are blessed with an opportunity to make choices.

I have found that defining my standards and prinicples, and putting them in written form to use as a personal reference guide to my daily living.

I use four categories:
VISION - MISSION – PHILOSOPHY - SYSTEMS

VISION:
And God said, Let there be Light.
And God saw the Light and that it was good;
And, He separated the Light from the darkness.
Genesis 1:3,4

You are the Light of the world.
A city on a hill cannot be hidden.
Matthew 5:14

With the purpose of shining my Light to
promote God's Goodness and Possibilities,
I will use, learn, and further develop
the many talents with which God has blessed me
to facilitate communication, and maximizing
the abilitiy to share love and compassion, in
order to support and encourage recovery through
positive personal growth and relationships.

PEOPLE WHO LIVE THROUGH TRANSPLANTS OR

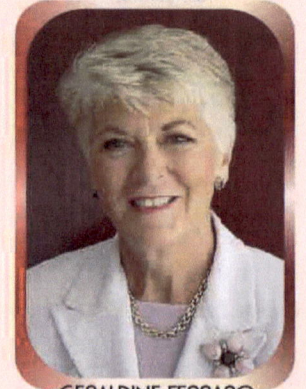

GERALDINE FERRARO
1935 - 2011

DISASTERS LIKE 9/11 ARE SURVIVORS.

(C) DAVIDWRIGHTLIVE.COM

MISSION:
Be Holy as I am Holy.
1 Peter 1:16
Believing I am a Holy child of God,
created in God's image, to shine His Light for good,
I bring my understanding of God's Will to earth using
the talents with which I have been blessed
to promote healing, acceptance, peace, love, and joy,
through my thoughts, words, and deeds.

PHILOSOPHY:
I can do all things through Him
who strengthens me.
Phillippians 4:13

Ask and it shall be given;
Seek and you shall find;
Knock and the door will be opened to you.
Matthew 7:7-11

With God in me, near me, and all around me,
all things are possible.

SYSTEMS:
In Him we live and move and have our being.
Acts 17:28

With scripture, prayer, God and the Holy Spirit within
as my foundation, while understanding the
teachings of Jesus Christ, Our Lord,
WILLINGLY,
I use my hands, feet, mouth, head, and heart to
promote my life's personal Vision, Mission, and Philosophy.

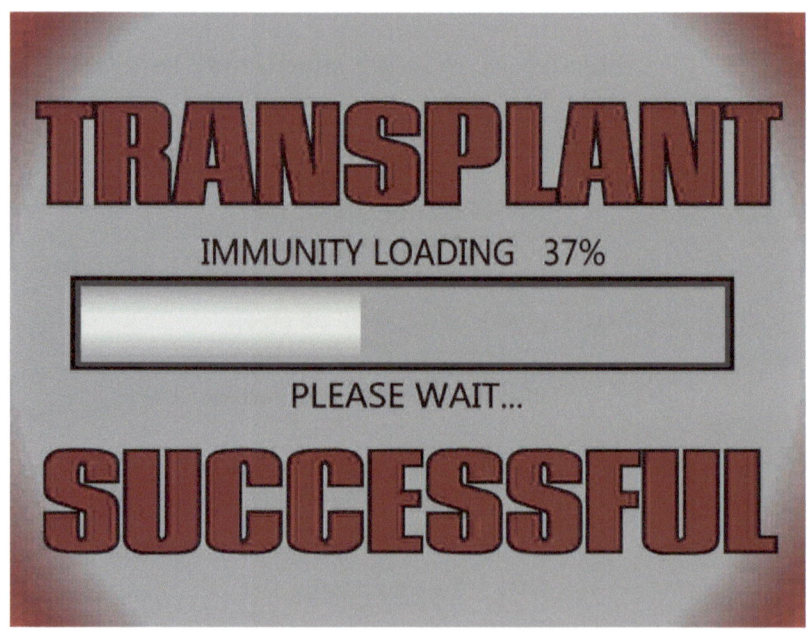

THE SURVIVOR
GETTING STARTED

GOAL SETTING

It is as simple as,
PLAN YOUR WORK – WORK YOUR PLAN.

If you listen to your Inner Voice, and understand
that God has a plan for you, for good – always,
and listen within for the ideas about where to start,
all will be revealed to you.

*Write them all down,
but then,
CHOOSE JUST ONE!*

You may have just one, or a hundred, as you start regaining real consciousness while the prescription medication is wearing off, but as you look at the ideas pouring forth, one will become the closest to your heart.

If you had nothing standing in your way today, but your recovery, which one would you choose?

*** _____ ***

WHY?

*** _____ ***

MISSION

Be Holy as I am Holy.
1 Peter 1:16

Believing I am a Holy child of God,
created in God's image,
to shine His Light for good,
I bring God's Will to earth using
the talents with which
I have been blessed
to promote healing, acceptance,
peace, love, and joy, through my
thoughts, words, and deeds.

(C) 2013 - DAVIDWRIGHTLIVE.COM

VISION-MISSION-PHILOSOPHY-SYSTEMS

CHOICES OF A SURVIVOR

As a survivor, you are surrounded by people who support your recovery and want only the best for you.

You got through it.

You are here – once again.

What better time to clear your mind, and focus first on your vision of what you can do next – LET THEM HELP YOU RECOVER!

With POSITIVE THOUGHTS and INTENTIONS, look WITHIN, and then WRITE DOWN what you want create – first, for you, using the gifts you have been given over a lifetime.

Even if you write down JUST ONE WORD – ALL OF A SUDDEN - you are on your way!

If you get stuck, stop, and rest.

With any goal, "JUST ONE" is the place to start.

Date:

VISION:

MISSION:

PHILOSOPHY:

SYSTEMS:

Come back to this page, and elaborate during your recovery as it starts to come together.

Keep track by dating each entry.

You'll be amazed later as you can see it growing over time – instead of just expecting the end result is instantaneous.

ALWAYS REMEMBER: GOD'S TIMING IS PERFECT!

PHILOSOPHY

I can do all things through
Him who strengthens me.
Phillippians 4:13

Ask and it shall be given;
Seek and you shall find;
Knock and the door
will be opened to you.
Matthew 7:7-11

With God in me, near me,
and all around me,
all things are possible.

(C) 2013 - DAVIDWRIGHTLIVE.COM

WHAT WERE
THE LESSONS LEARNED?

Yea, though I walk through the
Valley of the Shadow of Death...
Yup.
Been there?
Done that!
You've got the scar as the reminder.

Is there a *LESSON LEARNED* that
you could pass along to others?

Are there *LESSONS LEARNED* that,
with PRIDE, you can list out as
UNSHAKABLE
as you take the first steps
on your new journey?

*** _____ ***
*** _____ ***
*** _____ ***

WHY?

*** _____ ***
*** _____ ***
*** _____ ***

SYSTEMS

In Him we live and move
and have our being.
Acts 17:28

With scripture, prayer, and
God and the Holy Spirit within
as my foundation.

WILLINGLY
I use my hands, feet,
mouth, mind, and heart to
promote my life's personal
Vision, Mission, and Philosophy.

(C) 2013 - DAVIDWRIGHTLIVE.COM

RESOURCES AT HAND

SYSTEMS

Wherever you are reading this guide, you are living in a place where the abundance of the resources at hand have been provided by people all around you who believe in you, and want you to have a successful recovery.

The systems they have are all designed as cogs in the wheel of your individual life.

Within the Divine Plan that God has prepared for you, it is time for you to step up and paint the canvas in the way you want it to look.

Everyone around you is there to help you reach the result you want for you, and for those who will benefit by you being here.

There is "JUST ONE MORE THING" you have to do – today:

ASK!

Everyone with whom you interact during your recovery asks you questions according to their agenda – be it professional, or personal, and all are asked in sincerity.

It is time you did the same!

Set a goal to ask everyone who comes to see you, something other than, "How are you?" - ask *JUST ONE!*

The oldest questions in the book:

WHO-WHAT-WHERE-WHEN-WHY-HOW!

WHO do you know that... <insert something related to your vision> ...I could talk to about that?

WHAT do you think about...<insert your idea>?

WHERE would I find information about...<your idea>?

WHEN could you get back to me about... <your idea>?

WHY would people you know like to hear about...<your idea>?

HOW does that sound to you... <listening for a reaction!>?

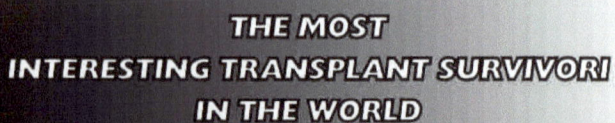

PRAYER IN RECOVERY
THE SACRED SILENCE

MEDITATION – TURNING WITHIN

After your successful transplant,
you alone are being given the opportunity
to make the upcoming changes one step at a time –
each step one day at a time.
In the sacred silence of meditation and prayer,
as you willingly look and listen within,
you will find answers you have never found before.

I will be reaching out to you as well.
This book was written as a result of the time I have spent
in the sacred silence of meditation and prayer.

I pray asking for you to be guided to
TURN WITHIN, LISTEN FOR THE INNER VOICE,
and to put your time to the
HIGHEST and BEST POSSIBLE USE.

Thank you for taking the time
to join me on my journey.

Let us thank God together in prayer.

FIND EVEN MORE
INTERESTING IDEAS
AT
BENNYPHISHERAREE.COM
by
Benny Phisheraree and David Fraser Wright

50 Weird Ideas
ISBN-13: 978-1492108603
ISBN-10: 149210860X

25 Weird Ideas
ISBN-13: 978-1492325598
ISBN-10: 1492325597

The Art of Karaoke
101 T-Shirt Designs
ISBN-13: 978-1492150299
ISBN-10: 1492150290

The Art of Karaoke
102 T-Shirt Designs
ISBN-13: 978-1492155591
ISBN-10: 1492155594

The Art of Karaoke
103 T-Shirt Designs
ISBN-13: 978-1492162797
ISBN-10: 1492162795

The Art of Karaoke
104 T-Shirt Designs
ISBN-13: 978-1492180210
ISBN-10: 1492180211

99 AA T-Shirt Designs Volume One
ISBN-13: 978-1492189367
ISBN-10: 1492189367

99 AA T-Shirt Designs Volume Two
ISBN-13: 978-1492214601
ISBN-10: 1492214604

Drunk On Power?
ISBN-13: 978-1492257257
ISBN-10: 1492257257

Drunk On Power, Again?
ISBN-13: 978-1492269670
ISBN-10: 1492269670

Nigeria 419 – 101 Reasons
ISBN-13: 978-1490992266
ISBN-10: 149099226X

Nigeria 419 – 102 Reasons
ISBN-13: 978-1491230657
ISBN-10: 1491230657

Nigeria 419 – 103 Reasons
ISBN-13: 978-1491285824
ISBN-10: 1491285826

TRANSPLANT: SUCCESSFUL!

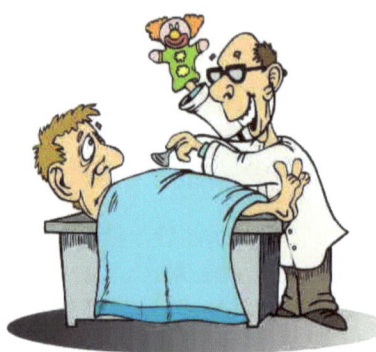

ALL OF A SUDDEN I CAN PLAY THE VIOLIN! WHAT IS THAT ALL ABOUT?

BY THE WAY...

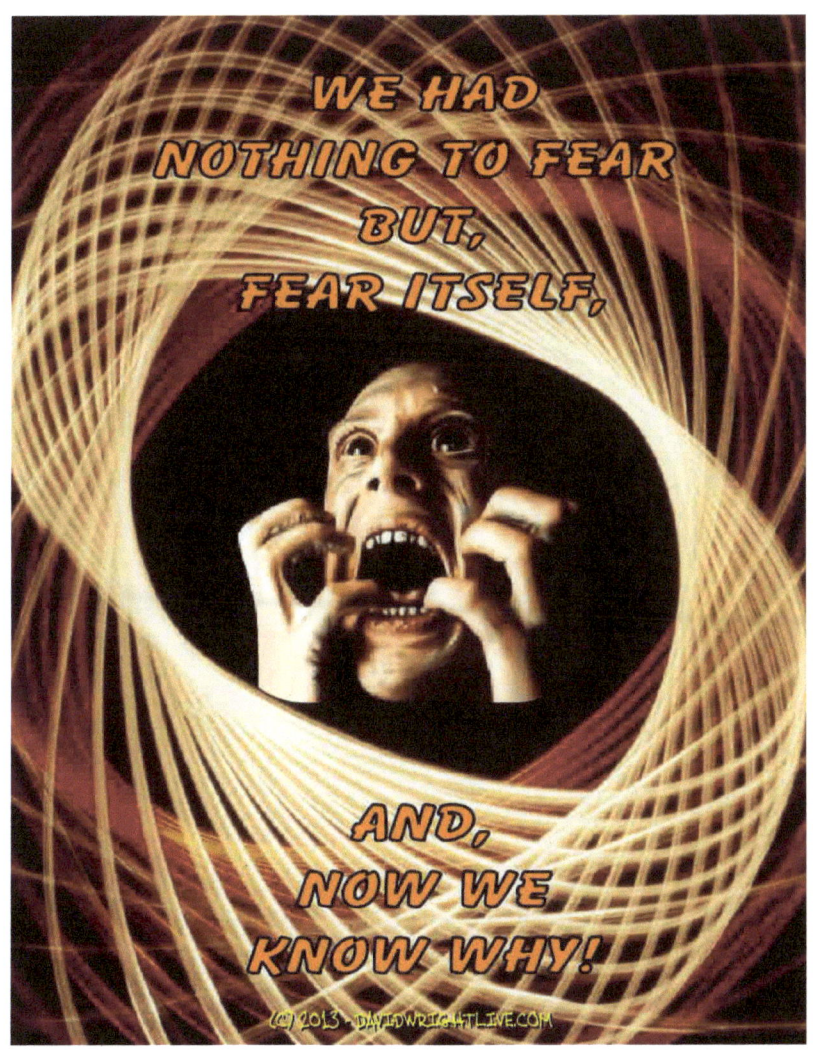

www.ingramcontent.com/pod-product-compliance
Lightning Source LLC
Chambersburg PA
CBHW040832180526
45159CB00001B/165